Enhance Your Health *with* FERMENTED FOODS

Warren Jefferson

live healthy now!

HEALTHY LIVING PUBLICATIONS
Summertown, Tennessee

Cover and interior design: Scattaregia Design

Healthy Living Publications,
a division of Book Publishing Company
PO Box 99
Summertown, TN 38483
888-260-8458
bookpubco.com

ISBN: 978-1-57067-323-8

20 19 18 17 16 15 1 2 3 4 5 6 7 8 9

Library of Congress Cataloging-in-Publication Data

Jefferson, Warren.
Enhance your health with fermented foods / Warren Jefferson.
pages cm
Includes bibliographical references.
ISBN 978-1-57067-323-8 (pbk.) -- ISBN 978-1-57067-873-8 (e-book)
1. Probiotics. 2. Fermented foods--Health aspects. I. Title.
RM666.P835J44 2015
613.2'6--dc23
2014046265

Printed on recycled paper

Book Publishing Company is a member of Green Press Initiative. We chose to print this title on paper with 100% post-consumer recycled content, processed without chlorine, which saved the following natural resources:

- 18 trees
- 563 pounds of solid waste
- 8,414 gallons of water
- 1,551 pounds of greenhouse gases
- 8 million BTU of energy

For more information on Green Press Initiative, visit www.greenpressinitiative.org. Environmental impact estimates were made using the Environmental Defense Fund Paper Calculator. For more information, visit papercalculator.org.

CONTENTS

Introduction

If you enjoy eating foods such as dill pickles, sauerkraut, and yogurt or sipping a glass of wine, you're experiencing the pleasures of fermented foods and beverages. At the same time, though you may not realize it, you're getting many important health benefits.

Humans have been consuming fermented foods and drink for at least ten thousand years. We know this because of the discovery in China of a large cache of pottery jars from the Neolithic period. Many of the jars contained a residue that turned out to be the ancient remnants of a fermented beverage made of grapes, honey, rice, and the fruit of the hawthorn tree. But it wasn't until about 150 years ago that scientists discovered that microscopic organisms called microbes were responsible for fermentation.

Microbes have populated the earth for at least 3,500 billion years, as evidenced by fossils found in rocks from that time. Microbes perform essential functions that maintain the health of the biosphere and all living creatures. They're also an integral part of the web of life and death, responsible for breaking down plant matter, dead animals, and waste products. The resulting end products are simple substances that then become the building blocks for other life.

Inside and out, our bodies are covered with microbes. We couldn't exist without the beneficial relationship we have with them. However, although we can't live without them, they can live without us quite well.

The microbes that inhabit our intestines are particularly important. The intestinal microbiota, as the flora in the intestines is called, is now considered an essential organ, just like the heart or liver. The microorganisms that make up the intestinal microbiota are involved in digestion, immune cell development, pathogen resistance, and other important body processes. Outside the body, some of the same microorganisms are key players in producing the myriad forms of fermented foods that nourish people throughout the world.

The fermentation of food is all about manipulating microorganisms to achieve a desired food product. A notable group of bacteria is lactic acid bacteria, which is responsible for producing the most fermented food in tons per year and the greatest variety of fermented foods, either independently or in concert with other microorganisms. Certain strains of lactic acid bacteria are the predominant species that make up intestinal flora, and they are included in most probiotic supplement formulas, which are used to boost the number of beneficial microbes in the digestive tract.

Microbes include bacteria, molds, and yeasts, many of which are beneficial and safe to consume. These microbes produce enzymes that are essential to the natural process of fermentation. Enzymes break down foods and other substances into simpler compounds and nutrients. Alcohol and acids are the two primary end products of fermentation, and since most of the microorganisms responsible for spoiling food cannot survive in alcoholic or acidic environments, fermentation is an effective and efficient method of food preservation. In addition, fermentation enhances food's nutritional value, increases its digestibility, and alters its aroma, flavor, and texture in agreeable ways.

It's easy to imagine how fermented foods found their way into human diets. In temperate and tropical regions, our early ancestors would surely have come upon rotting or fermenting fruits and vegetation. Through trial and error, they would have discovered that some were edible and pleasing to the palate. They also would have observed that drinking the juice of fermenting fruit produced profound mind-altering effects—it would get them high—and so people were evermore hooked on fermented drinks. Some archaeologists theorize that one of the main reasons early humans settled down and started to farm was to ensure a constant supply of alcoholic beverages. In fact, in addition to bread, wine and beer are thought to be the first fermented products made by man.

Fermented foods are consumed worldwide, and every region has its own particular version, determined by the raw materials available and the natural microbes living there. For example, in North America, we're familiar with beer, cucumber pickles, hard cider, sauerkraut, and wine, but countless different kinds of fermented foods and beverages are produced around the world. Fermented foods play a significant role in helping to meet the nutritional needs of the earth's population; in fact, fermented foods account for almost one-third of all food consumed globally.

In the following pages you'll learn about the different types of fermented foods from around the world and the microbes that produce them. You'll also discover the many benefits of fermented foods and some potential concerns you should be aware of. And you'll find simple instructions for how to easily make some fermented products, such as cucumber pickles, rejuvelac, and sauerkraut, at home.

In the past twenty-five years there has been renewed interest in fermented food products and their nutritional and therapeutic properties. Developments in microbiology and fermentation technology continue to evolve. New techniques, such as using more concentrated mediums, result in higher yields and rapid production that relies on less oxygen. The ancient technique of fermentation is, at long last, becoming new and improved, although traditional methods remain as successful as ever.

So read on. You're about to enter the amazing world of microbes and delicious fermented foods.

A Fermented Superstar: Sauerkraut

Sauerkraut is an enzyme-rich living food containing millions of friendly bacteria. It's low in calories, highly nutritious, and contains vitamins B and C. For a sauerkraut recipe, see page 28. When buying commercially produced sauerkraut, choose a brand that's not pasteurized. The high temperatures reached during pasteurization kill the friendly bacteria.

Benefits of Fermented Foods and Beverages

Many advantages come from eating fermented foods. We know about some of them, but there are almost certainly many more we don't know about or are just getting indications of. Some of the known health benefits come from eating fermented foods, such as sauerkraut, that contain live cultures (see box, previous page). Other benefits come from consuming foods or beverages that are the products of fermentation but no longer contain live cultures. These include alcoholic drinks, soy sauce, and tempeh.

Fermentation imparts appealing and unique aromas, flavors, and textures to a food or beverage. It makes food more digestible by breaking down carbohydrates, fats, and proteins—in a sense, by predigesting food. And it enhances the nutritional value of foods by increasing the concentrations of certain phytochemicals and vitamins. Fermentation has also been shown to eliminate toxins and antinutrients, which interfere with absorption or advantageous functions, in some foods.

Fermented foods increase and add diversity to the population of intestinal flora and produce substances that benefit the nervous system and normalize blood pressure. It has been found that a number of lactic acid bacteria produce antibiotics and bacteriocins, which are antibiotics made by bacteria. Antibiotics can be helpful because they kill harmful bacteria. Molds can also produce antibiotics. Probiotics, or helpful microorganisms, naturally occur in fermented foods and can enhance the gut flora. In addition, compounds in fermented foods protect against the development of some cancers. Studies involving mice have shown that certain fermented foods possess anticancer and anti-inflammatory properties.

Research in nutritional psychiatry has indicated a connection between the brain and intestinal flora. For example, a balanced and healthy intestinal flora has been shown to help reduce depression and anxiety.

Alcohol is a fermented substance with known health advantages as well as disadvantages. Alcohol consumption has been linked with depression, for instance. However, small amounts can be beneficial, as noted in a study published in the *Journal of Physiological Anthropology* in 2014: "When consumed in modest amounts (.18 to .53 ounces or 5 to 15 g per day) as part of traditional dietary practices, alcohol (red wine in particular) has been associated with a lower risk of depression. Indeed, light to moderate alcohol consumption has also been associated with lower systemic inflammation." So enjoy your red wine, beer, or whiskey, but in moderation.

While science continues to help us understand the many ways that consuming fermented items can boost specific aspects of health, these products provide much more global advantages. Access to adequate, nutritious food is limited for millions of people in countries with developing economies. Notably, fermented foods help fill the gap in regions where some types of agricultural waste are converted into palatable and nourishing consumables. For instance, an Indonesian food called *ontjom* is made from the by-products of peanut and coconut processing. And in some areas where pineapples are grown and processed, pineapple peels are fermented and made into a light pineapple-flavored vinegar. Palm wine produced in western Africa is high in vitamin B_{12}, and sorghum beer produced in southern Africa contains riboflavin and nicotinic acid, important for people subsisting mainly on a diet of corn.

Other healthful fermented items are made from raw materials that are plentiful in certain areas. *Pulque*, the national drink of Mexico, plays an important role in the nutrition of low-income people. Pulque is a milky, acidic, and slightly foamy beverage thought to have been introduced by the Aztecs. It has an alcohol content of 6 to 7 percent, and the spirits mescal and tequila are made from it.

Pulque is made by fermenting the juice of various agave cacti. Fermentation occurs naturally in response to the presence of wild yeasts. *Leuconostoc*, a genus of bacteria, give the pulque its characteristic viscosity. Fermentation increases the drink's nutritional value by significantly boosting the amount of the vitamins, niacin, riboflavin, and thiamine that it contains.

Another important benefit of fermentation for people in poorer countries is that fermented foods require less cooking or no cooking at all, saving precious fuel. As an example, consider soybeans and tempeh. Soybeans normally require four to five hours of cooking time, but tempeh, a food made from fermented soybeans, requires only fifteen minutes. Sauerkraut and pickled vegetables require no cooking at all. Fermentation is an inexpensive and energy-efficient way to preserve perishable food as opposed to other methods, such as canning, drying, and freezing. The greatest advantage of all may be that fermentation maintains the live beneficial microorganisms in foods, whereas other types of preservation diminish or destroy them.

Possible Adverse Reactions to Eating Fermented Foods

Fermented foods have a very good safety record throughout the world. The benefits clearly outweigh the dangers. But like any other type of food preservation, if fermentation is not done correctly, the food will spoil.

Fermented foods may be problematic for individuals with specific conditions or sensitivities. For example, if you have candida or thrush, or if you're allergic to mold, use caution when eating fermented foods containing molds and yeasts, which can aggravate these conditions. In addition, some fermented items, such as cheese and wine, are naturally high in histamine and could cause an allergic response in people who are sensitive to this compound.

Rarely, certain fermented foods have prompted regional health concerns. A study in the *British Journal of Cancer* in 2009 showed a twofold increase in esophageal cancer in a population in northern China; this increase was attributed to the consumption of fermented vegetables. The population consumed pickled vegetables every day for nine to twelve months each year. It's thought that harmful, indigenous microorganisms (perhaps fungi) were able to grow in the pickled vegetables and produce compounds with carcinogenic properties.

History of Fermented Foods and Drinks

The documented use of fermented foods goes back to Neolithic times, but some of the first writings we have on food fermentation are by the Roman scholar Pliny the Elder (AD 23–79). In his encyclopedic work *Natural History*, he gives us the best methods for turning grape juice into wine and for preventing it from turning sour.

Indeed, fermentation has long been especially valued for its role in creating intoxicating drinks. Fermented alcoholic beverages have been cultivated and consumed by most, if not all, cultures throughout history, and they have played a key role in the development of these cultures and their technology. The consumption of fermented beverages was an integral part of secular and religious ceremonies, harvests and other celebrations, and even somber life events.

Vegetable fermentation is thought to have originated in Asia around two thousand years ago. During the construction of the Great Wall of China in the third century BC, workers were fed fermented vegetables, such as cabbages, cucumbers, radishes, and turnips.

Fermented cereals, dairy products, meats and seafood, and vegetables were a significant part of the diet of our early ancestors, and as agriculture developed, so did fermentation techniques. In medieval Europe, fermented foods were consumed as part of the daily diet. In the eighteenth century, British explorer and captain James Cook kept his men free of scurvy by feeding them sauerkraut during their around-the-world sailing voyage.

The production of fermented food and beverages was well established by modern times, but little was known about how the process actually worked. Anton van Leeuwenhoek and Robert Hooke are credited with the discovery of microorganisms (protozoa and yeast) in 1675, which was possible with the use of the newly invented microscope. Protozoa were obviously alive, but yeast didn't seem to display any movement. No connection was made between the existence of these microscopic organisms and the well-known phenomenon of fermentation, however, for 150 years.

Around 1837 it was discovered that yeast was a living organism. The discovery of bacteria soon followed. In 1857 Louis Pasteur showed that fermentation was caused by living organisms and was not a chemical reaction. In 1860 he showed that bacteria soured milk; ten years later he presented his germ theory and soon after developed the process of pasteurization. It was during this period that he published his famous paper "Studies in Fermentation," in which he showed that specific microorganisms cause certain types of fermentation and end products.

In 1897 the German chemist Eduard Buchner discovered that fermentation did not require living organisms. He first used the term "enzymes" to apply to all ferments and soon discovered that enzymes are not living microorganisms but are produced by them. Enzymes are the agents, or catalysts, that make fermentation possible. Buchner won the Nobel Prize in 1907 for his biochemical investigations and discovery of non-cellular fermentation. In 1908, Russian biologist Elie Metchnikoff proposed that fermented dairy products have beneficial properties.

Fermented foods were first cultivated in individual households and later their production became a cottage industry. Today certain fermented foods and beverages are mass produced, but in less industrialized nations, most fermented foods are still made in the small-scale, traditional way.

Microorganisms

Microorganisms are the most abundant life form on Earth in terms of biomass and the number of species. In fact, the world's microorganisms outweigh all other living creatures on the planet combined! Microorganisms have inhabited the planet for at least 3,500 billion years, and they were the only life form for most of that time. Around 2,800 billion years ago, a very special microorganism called blue-green algae, or cyanobacteria, appeared. This was an important development for life on Earth, for these algae were the first microorganisms that could perform photosynthesis, the use of the sun's energy to create oxygen. They're thought to be responsible for raising the oxygen in the earth's atmosphere from 1 percent to the current level of 21 percent, making it possible for more complex life forms to evolve.

Microorganisms live in every habitat in the biosphere, including the most extreme environments of cold, heat, and dryness. They live in oceans, rocks, snow, and soil, as well as on and in the bodies of animals, humans, and plants. Bacteria come in a wide variety of shapes and sizes and can live in pairs, chains, or clusters.

Beneficial Effects of Microorganisms

Microorganisms metabolize organic matter by consuming it, effectively recycling the matter by breaking it down into primary elements, such as carbon, nitrogen, and oxygen. These elements in turn serve as the building blocks for other life. Microorganisms can break down every naturally occurring organic compound and some inorganic compounds as well. If they were to disappear today, the earth would quickly become a gigantic refuse dump, and all advanced life forms would soon die off.

Different types of microorganisms provide different essential functions. These include the following:

Nitrogen fixation. The process of nitrogen fixation occurs when bacteria capture nitrogen from the atmosphere and convert it to ammonia that can be used by plants and animals. These bacteria live in dependent and cooperative, or symbiotic, associations with plants and add nitrogen to the soil. Some live not in plants but in soil and water habitats.

Oxygenic photosynthesis. Algae, cyanobacteria, and plants perform oxygenic photosynthesis, an essential process that results in the production of oxygen in the atmosphere. It's estimated that algae and cyanobacteria produce at least half this oxygen; terrestrial plants produce the rest.

Primary production. Primary production depends on the synthesis of carbon dioxide and the process of photosynthesis. Photosynthetic microorganisms floating in the sea take up carbon dioxide in the atmosphere and convert it to organic cellular material, a process called carbon fixation. These unicellular organisms, floating in the sea, account for almost half the carbon fixation that takes place on the planet; terrestrial plants account for the rest. Combined, these organisms and plants provide the carbon required for the synthesis of cell material for more complex forms of life.

The cyanobacterium *Synechococcus* is an exceptional species and one of the most important found in marine habitats. This microorganism does it all—nitrogen fixation, oxygenic photosynthesis, and primary production—accounting for almost 25 percent of the primary production in a typical marine habitat.

Microbiota: Intestinal Flora

There are more than 100 trillion microbial cells in and on the human body. They're called the normal human flora, or microbiota, and consist of more than ten thousand species of microorganisms. The cells in the microbiota outnumber human cells ten to one and have over eight million unique genes as compared to the human set of about 22,000. Many scientists consider the human microbiota to be an acquired organ, on par with the other organs of the body, because of the complexity and number of life processes it performs and the important part it plays in human health and disease. For example, the gut flora is believed to be involved in digestion, immune cell development, dental health, pathogen resistance, and other processes. The microbiota clearly plays a critical role in human survival.

The large intestine of a healthy adult contains trillions of microorganisms. The gut flora is made up of five hundred different species of bacteria, although 99 percent is composed of just thirty to forty species. This mass of microorganisms can weigh as much as 2.2 pounds (1 kg), and these microorganisms make up about 50 percent of fecal mass.

Each person feeds his or her own gut flora through diet and must provide about 250 calories of carbohydrates per day just to keep the bacteria in the gut flora alive. Most of these bacteria are beneficial or harmless, but some cause disease. Each species prefers specific nutrients. Most of the bacteria that are beneficial to the host feed on plant-based carbohydrates, while most bacteria that cause disease in the host feed on animal protein and processed foods.

An imbalance between good and bad bacteria can lead to a number of health problems. Functional bowel disorders; inflammatory bowel diseases and other immune-mediated inflammatory diseases, such as allergies and celiac disease; metabolic conditions, such as type 2 diabetes; and even mental conditions, such as autism and depression, are all linked to an imbalance in the gut microbiota.

Among healthy adults, the composition of the gut flora varies. One-third of the makeup is quite similar from person to person, but two-thirds of the composition is unique to the individual, like fingerprints. The types of microorganisms that thrive in a person's gut flora are determined by diet, environment, age, and other factors. And the composition of the gut flora continues to evolve throughout a person's life, so the gut flora of an older person is different from the flora they had when young.

Our gut flora begins developing at birth, and possibly before. It has long been believed that because of the placental barrier, a fetus is sterile in the uterus and has no microbiota before birth. But evidence is beginning to show that babies acquire their initial inoculum of microbiota from the mother in the womb, before birth. A baby's microbiota is further enhanced during the birth process and by kissing, fondling, and breastfeeding. In just forty-eight hours, it's quite well established. By age three, a child's gut flora is fully developed and similar to an adult's.

The exact relationship between people and their gut flora isn't well understood, but it's thought to be interactive and dynamic rather than static and indifferent. The association between a human host and friendly bacteria is for the most part mutualistic, that is, beneficial. The gut flora receives nutrients, a hospitable environment, and transport as the host goes about daily activities. The host receives some nutritional and digestive benefits, stimulation of the immune system, and protection against invasion from pathogenic microbes.

Beneficial Effects

Certain bacteria in the gut are known to perform the following beneficial tasks:

- Stimulate the production of natural antibodies.
- Prevent colonization of pathogens by competing for nutrients and colony sites.
- Inhibit or kill invasive species of harmful bacteria through the production of antibacterial and antifungal substances.
- Synthesize and excrete vitamins K and B, vitamins that can be used by the host.

The beneficial effects listed here are taken from studies of germ-free animals (mice and hamsters) that were not colonized with normal flora as compared to animals that were colonized with normal flora. Note that the beneficial bacteria also stimulated the development of certain tissues in the gastrointestinal tracts of the animals with normal flora, whereas the germ-free animals had poor development of these tissues.

Harmful Effects

Some bacteria are parasites that live at the expense of their host. And pathogenic microbes living in the gut flora are capable of producing disease in the host. In these situations, the host has a weakness or diminishment of defenses, and the pathogen can multiply and eventually cause infection.

The gut flora can become out of balance, a condition called dysbiosis. This imbalance can lead to a variety of health problems, such as allergies, diabetes, functional bowel disorders, inflammatory bowel disease, and obesity.

Certain bacteria in the gut are known to perform the following harmful actions:

- Allow gut flora to supply essential growth factors for certain disease-causing, or pathogenic, microbes.
- Promote antibiotic resistance when a resistant bacterium develops and shares its resistance with a pathogen that would normally be killed by an antibiotic drug.
- Compete with the host for nutrients. Specifically, a germ-free host grows more rapidly than one with a healthy microbiota. This is why factory-farmed animals that are given antibiotics grow more rapidly, and as a result can go to market at a younger age than animals that aren't given antibiotics.
- Transfer to other hosts through coughing, sneezing, and other mechanisms and develop into infections.
- Change as the result of poor nutrition or antibiotic use and lead to gastrointestinal disease.
- Produce carcinogenic metabolites that have been associated with colon cancer.
- Colonize and lead to serious disease. For example, colonies of the pathogenic bacterium *Helicobacter pylori* cause gastric ulcers and may be the cause of gastric and duodenal cancer.

Like the beneficial effects listed previously, the harmful effects described here are taken from studies of germ-free animals (mice and hamsters) that were not colonized with normal flora as compared to animals that were colonized with normal flora.

Basic Principles of Food Fermentation

Food fermentation is a natural chemical process that is all about microbes and how to make them work to our advantage to produce a desired food product. The trick is to control the process so only the desired bacteria, molds, or yeasts grow on the substance that feeds them, which is known as the substrate. The substrate is typically alcoholic or acidic because most organisms that cause foods to spoil cannot survive in these environments. As the desirable organisms grow, they compete for available nutrients with organisms that cause spoilage and at the same time create a hostile environment that suppresses the spoilers.

Fermentation is the method used to produce a large variety of food products, but the microbes that give rise to these foods come from only six genera, or types, of bacteria, eight genera of molds, and five genera of yeasts. These three groups of microorganisms are naturally and widely distributed throughout our environment and are important to the food industry.

In the process of fermentation, the microorganisms grown on the substrate produce enzymes that break down the food in the substrate into more easily digested compounds and nutrients. The enzymes chemically break down the food with water, a process known as hydrolysis. As a result, proteins are converted into amino acids, carbohydrates into simple sugars, and fats into free fatty acids. In addition, alcohol, carbon dioxide, and other gases are generated as by-products. The final food product has enhanced nutritional value along with flavors, aromas, and textures that are pleasing to the palate.

Types of Fermenting Organisms

Bacteria, molds, and yeasts are essential for fermentation. Most food fermentation is the result of two or more microorganisms working either together or in sequence. An example is the production of vinegar, which is a mixed fermentation of yeast and bacteria. First, yeasts convert the sugar in the substrate (fruit juice) into alcohol, then *Acetobacter* bacteria convert the alcohol into acetic acid and water.

Bacteria. There are several families of bacteria present in food. Most are involved in food spoilage, but some are beneficial. The most important bacteria in desirable food fermentation are from the Lactobacillaceae family, which produces lactic acid from carbohydrates as the end product of fermentation. These bacteria are anaerobic, meaning they grow in the absence of oxygen. Sauerkraut is a prime example of a fermented food that grows in the absence of oxygen.

Other important bacteria in food fermentation are from the genus *Acetobacter*. These bacteria convert alcohol to acetic acid and water. Vinegar is an excellent example of a product resulting from this conversion.

Molds. The robust genus *Aspergillus* is a common food spoiler that can develop in strong concentrations of salt or sugar. Molds can grow on most foods, and they produce the greatest number and diversity of enzymes.

Molds are essential in the production of cheese, with certain species imparting unique, palate-pleasing flavors and textures. For instance, *Penicillium roqueforti*, which is in the same family as *Aspergillus,* is involved in the making of Roquefort, Stilton, and other blue cheeses. The molds are aerobic, meaning they require free oxygen to grow. Molds are not very active in the fermentation of fruits and vegetables.

Yeasts. The most important yeasts in desirable food fermentation are from the genus *Saccharomyces*, especially the species *S. cerevisiae*, which is used in the production of bread and alcoholic beverages.

Controlling the Growth and Activity of Fermentation

In addition to nutrient content, there are five other factors that can control microbes in foods. These are moisture, the availability of oxygen, temperature, hydrogen ion concentration (pH), and inhibitors.

Moisture

Moisture is necessary for cells to grow and metabolize. Drying and freezing affects the moisture available to microbial cells. Two types of water are available to cells: bound water and free water. Bound water is the water within the cell wall and is essential for all biological processes within the cell. Free water is the water around the cells and is essential for the functioning of microorganisms. When free water is removed, the growth and activity of most microorganisms can be controlled.

The amount of water in a food product determines the amount of water available to microorganisms and is referred to as the water activity. The water activity scale extends from 0 (bone dry) to 1 (pure water). Bacteria need more water than yeasts, and yeasts require more water than molds. Most microbial activity is inhibited at a water activity level below 0.6. Most bacteria are inhibited below 0.9, yeasts below 0.8, and molds below 0.7. The water activity level of a food product can be changed by decreasing the free water available through drying or freezing or by adding salt or sugar. A change in the water activity level can encourage the growth of beneficial microorganisms and discourage the growth of spoilage microorganisms.

Oxygen

Microbiologists broadly classify microorganisms into two groups: aerobic and anaerobic. Aerobic microorganisms grow in the presence of free oxygen; anaerobic microorganisms grow in the absence of free oxygen. Some microorganisms can metabolize the oxygen that is bound to the substrate.

Temperature

Temperature has an effect on the growth and activity of microorganisms. At high temperatures, microorganisms are destroyed (as occurs when food is cooked), and at low temperatures, microorganism activity is greatly reduced or suspended (as occurs when food is frozen). Microorganisms can be further classified by type according to their temperature preference:

- Psychrophilic microorganisms grow in a minimum temperature of 32 to 41 degrees F (0 to 5 degrees C), with optimum growth at 59 to 68 degrees F (15 to 20 degrees C) and a maximum temperature of 86 degrees F (30 degrees C).

- Mesophilic microorganisms grow at a minimum temperature of 50 to 77 degrees F (10 to 25 degrees C), with optimum growth at 86 to 104 degrees F (30 to 40 degrees C) and a maximum temperature of 122 degrees F (50 degrees C).
- Thermophilic microorganisms grow in a minimum temperature of 77 to 113 degrees F (25 to 45 degrees C), with optimum growth at 122 to 131 degrees F (50 to 55 degrees C) and a maximum temperature of 194 degrees F (90 degrees C).

Hydrogen Ion Concentration, or pH

Manipulating a food or substrate to make it more acidic or more alkaline affects fermentation. The numerals 0 to 14 are used to define how acidic or alkaline a substance is, and this indicator is commonly known as the pH. Altering the pH of a food during fermentation is a very effective way to discourage spoilage microorganisms. Most bacteria favor a neutral pH, around 7. Yeasts favor a pH range of 4 to 4.5. Molds favor a pH of 2 to 8.5 but prefer a pH of 4.6 or lower—an acidic environment. High-acid foods, those with a pH of 4.6 or lower, will inhibit the growth of most bacteria. The exceptions are the acid-tolerant bacteria species *Lactobacillus* and *Streptococcus* that are used in dairy and vegetable fermentations. A food with a pH above 4.6 is a low-acid food and will not inhibit the growth of spoilage bacteria.

Inhibitors

Chemical compounds, such as a strong acid or alkaline, a concentrated salt, or an organic solvent, are used to inhibit the growth and activity of microorganisms. These compounds work by preventing the cells from metabolizing, denaturing the protein in the cells, or physically damaging the cells. Such functions cause the microbial action to cease.

Types of Fermentation

The fermented foods and beverages we consume are the result of lactic acid fermentation, acetic acid and vinegar fermentation, alkaline fermentation, and alcoholic fermentation. The differences are defined by the types of microorganisms, foods, and substrates involved. While these terms seem long and scientific, the fact remains that making fermented foods is easily done at home. Several recipes in this section will give you a chance to do just that.

Although this section concentrates on lactic acid fermentation and acetic acid and vinegar fermentation, it's worth noting other popular foods, drinks, and seasonings that result from alkaline fermentation and alcoholic fermentation. Alkaline fermentation, for example, relies on bacteria to produce primarily condiments from available foods, such as seeds and beans. Examples of these items, which provide not only taste but also nutrition, are natto, a Japanese breakfast food made from soybeans, and *ogiri*, an African condiment made from melon seeds.

Even if fermented foods aren't familiar to you, fermented alcoholic beverages probably are. Indeed, they've been popular the world over for thousands of years and have been resourcefully created from the raw materials at hand. Examples of regional fermented alcoholic drinks and the raw materials used to make them are Japanese sake made from rice; Mexican pulque from agave cactus; Ethiopian *tej*, a beer made from honey and grain; and a Nigerian beer called *pito* that's fermented from millet or sorghum.

Lactic Acid Bacteria and Lactic Acid Fermentation

Lactic acid bacteria, which are wild and widely distributed in nature, are among the most important microorganisms used in food fermentation. They are the same bacteria found in human mucous membranes and in the gut as a part of the microbiota.

The word "lactic" is derived from the Latin word for milk, and fermented, or sour, milk was probably the first lactic acid fermented food used by humans. Lactic acid fermentation is responsible for producing and preserving a large variety of different foods in vast quantities. Some typical North American foods that are produced using lactic acid bacteria include cheese, cucumber pickles, cultured butter, olives, sauerkraut, sour cream, and yogurt.

Lactic acid bacteria obtain their energy from the metabolism of sugar, so they can be used only in the production of foods that contain sugars. They convert the sugars in the food or substrate into lactic acid, which makes the environment too acidic for spoilage microbes to get established. This process also generates carbon dioxide, which replaces the oxygen, creating an anaerobic environment that further deters the development of many spoilage bacteria.

Most lactic acid bacteria live freely or in a mutually beneficial association with animals and humans. They are found in raw milk, on the surface of vegetables, and on decaying plant material. Because of these beneficial bacteria, raw milk will rapidly ferment at room temperature and is safe to use in recipes. If the watery liquid, known as whey, that forms after the milk sours is allowed to evaporate, the remaining curds will make a simple, natural cheese.

Why does this natural fermentation happen in raw milk? Cows feed on grass, and grass is covered with lactic acid bacteria. When a cow digests the grass, these bacteria are transferred to the cow's milk. Some strains are also picked up from the cow's intestinal microbiota.

Lactic acid bacteria are found naturally on the skins of vegetables and fruit. The white film found on fresh cucumbers, grapes, and plums, for example, indicates the presence of lactic acid bacteria. However, whey is typically added to most fermenting vegetables to provide nutrients for the bacteria and help the fermentation process get started. There are exceptions, however; for example, whey is not usually needed for cabbage and cucumber fermentation.

Not all lactic acid bacteria are useful in fermentation or beneficial to humans. Some can spoil beer, wine, and processed meats. Others are opportunistic pathogens and can cause disease. For instance, *Streptococcus pyogenes* causes strep throat, pneumonia, and scarlet fever. *Streptococcus pneumoniae* causes meningitis and other diseases. In addition, some oral streptococci contribute to dental cavities.

Lactic acid fermentation of vegetables requires only four elements. These include salt to draw out the vegetable juices at the beginning of the process, the proper temperature, an anaerobic environment, and a weight that submerges the food in the salt water and extracts liquid from the vegetable. The process can be very low-tech.

Microbes Involved in Lactic Acid Fermentation

Bacteria that are commonly used for the lactic acid fermentation of food include the following:

- *Bifidobacterium bifidum*
- *Lactobacillus acidophilus*
- *Lactobacillus brevis*
- *Lactobacillus bulgaricus*
- *Lactobacillus plantarum*
- *Leuconostoc citrovorum*
- *Leuconostoc mesenteroides*
- *Pediococcus cerevisiae*
- *Streptococcus lactis*
- *Streptococcus thermophilus*

Common Lactic Acid Fermented Foods and Drinks

Many of the foods and beverages produced by lactic acid fermentation are enthusiastically embraced staples, at least somewhere in the world. They may vary from region to region, but the popularity of such foods as bread, dairy products, pickled vegetables, and sauerkraut can't be denied. They range from kefir, a yogurt drink from the Caucasus, and olives from southern Europe to the exotically flavored mixed vegetable pickles of Southeast Asia and a Ghanian fermented corn dough, kenkey. Other specialties, such as the beverages Beet Kvass (page 29) and Rejuvelac (page 30), have long histories but are not as widely known.

Cucumber Pickles

Pickled cucumbers are produced and eaten around the world and are easy to make in the home kitchen. The cucumbers are fermented in a strong solution of salt and water, or brine, that draws sugar and water out of the vegetables, weakening the salt concentration. As a result, salt needs to be added to the brine periodically while the cucumbers ferment.

As the fermentation progresses, the cucumber skins change from bright green to dark olive green, and the cucumber flesh becomes translucent and waxy looking as air is forced out of the cells. As the cucumbers absorb the salt, they no longer float to the surface of the brine. During the first stage of fermentation, salt-tolerant *Leuconostoc mesenteroides* bacteria predominate. At this stage, the brine looks cloudy. During the final stage, *Lactobacillus* bacteria take over. Most commercial pickles are pasteurized and don't contain these healthful, live microorganisms.

Cucumber Pickles

Fermented pickles are a low-calorie food rich in vitamin K but also high in sodium, so they should be eaten in moderation. Herbs and spices, such as dried dill weed and peppercorns, can be added to the brine to enhance the pickles' flavor.

1 gallon (4 L) filtered water
8 ounces (227 g) table salt or sea salt, or 10 ounces (284 g) kosher salt
Pickling cucumbers, washed and ends trimmed (the number needed will depend on the size of the pickles and the jar used)
Dried dill weed (optional)
Peppercorns (optional)

To make a brine, pour the water into a large bowl or pitcher and stir the salt into the water until diluted.

Pack the cucumbers in a sterilized widemouthed glass jar and add dill weed and peppercorns if desired. Cover with the brine. Top with a food-grade weight (available from a fermentation supply company; see Sources, page 46) or sanitized stone to keep the cucumbers completely submerged in the brine.

Cover the mouth of the jar with a muslin cloth and let sit in a cool, dark place. Fermentation starts when bubbles of carbon dioxide begin to form and break through the surface of the brine. After 1 or 2 days, stir the brine to redistribute the salt. Fermentation is complete when the bubbling ceases, usually in 1 to 4 weeks, depending on the ambient temperature. The optimum temperature for fermentation is 84 to 89 degrees F (29 to 32 degrees C).

Stored in a sealed jar in the refrigerator, Cucumber Pickles will keep for 6 months.

Kimchi

Kimchi is a staple in Korea, where daily consumption is estimated to be about 1 cup (250 ml) per person. Cabbage and other vegetables are chopped and soaked in a salt solution of 8 to 15 percent for two to seven hours to increase the salt content of the vegetables. After they are rinsed and drained, the vegetables are mixed with salt, spices, and flavorings and allowed to ferment. The important microorganisms for kimchi fermentation are *Lactobacillus brevis, Lactobacillus plantarum, Leuconostoc mesenteroides, Pediococcus pentosaceus*, and *Streptococcus faecalis*. The final product can be kept for several weeks if refrigerated but spoils rapidly if stored under warm conditions.

Dairy Products

Popular fermented dairy products include cheese, kefir, and yogurt. When cheese is fermented, many different microorganisms are used to transform the milk from cows, goats, and sheep, and a coagulant is often added to make the milk clot. Specific microbial cultures are chosen for the different aromas, flavors, and textures they impart to the finished product. For instance, the pungent smell and flavor of Roquefort cheese is derived in part from the bacteria *Penicillium roqueforti.* Cheese also can be made without dairy milk; one plant-based alternative used to make vegan cheese is cashew milk.

Kefir is a tangy, slightly alcoholic, drinkable yogurt that can be made with raw cow's or goat's milk. It contains strains of bacteria that give it a unique taste. The principal species used to make kefir are the bacteria *Lactobacillus brevis* and the yeasts *Saccharomyces kefir and Torula kefir.*

Yogurt is the end result when bacteria are added to pasteurized raw milk. The two primary strains of bacteria used are *Lactobacillus bulgaricus* and *Streptococcus thermophilus*, although others are sometimes used. During fermentation, the sugar, or lactose, in the milk is changed to lactic acid. Because yogurt is easier to digest than milk, it may be a suitable food for lactose-intolerant people.

Sauerkraut

Sauerkraut has been made since classical times and is popular in Europe and North America. It's a low-calorie food that's relatively easy to produce in the home kitchen. During fermentation, salt-tolerant *Lactobacillus* bacteria feed on sugars in the cabbage and produce lactic acid.

Sauerkraut fermentation involves three stages during which different species of lactic acid bacteria dominate. In the first stage, *Leuconostoc mesenteroides* bacteria grow, producing lactic acid, carbon dioxide, and a little acetic acid. The carbon dioxide flushes out any oxygen, creating an anaerobic environment.

In the second stage, *Leuconostoc mesenteroides* bacteria slow down and begin to die off, and *Lactobacillus plantarum and L. cucumeris* bacteria take over, producing more lactic acid and carbon dioxide, until a pH level of 1.5 to 2 percent is reached.

Lactobacillus plantarum and L. cucumeris bacteria die off during the third stage, and *Lactobacillus brevis and L. pentoacetius* take over, producing even more lactic acid and lowering the pH to 2 to 2.5 percent. At this point, carbon dioxide bubbling ceases and the fermentation process is complete.

Some people use starter cultures to ensure consistent quality and speed up the process rather than rely on the work of naturally occurring wild bacteria. A starter culture is some type of medium, such as a grain or liquid, that is already colonized with the desired organisms. The bacteria *Streptococcus lactis*, for example, is used as a starter for sauerkraut and some dairy products, with good results. These bacteria efficiently initiate fermentation but quickly die off, and the *Leuconostoc mesenteroides* bacteria take over. When making sauerkraut, however, using juice from a previous batch as a starter is not recommended.

Most commercial sauerkraut is pasteurized and doesn't contain live microorganisms. Getting the health benefits afforded by consuming these beneficial microbes is the point of making sauerkraut at home. But keep in mind that sauerkraut can be spoiled by a number of factors, such as not keeping the fermenting cabbage completely submerged in the brine, improper salting, and temperature variations. One or more of these conditions can allow undesirable organisms to grow and ruin a batch, resulting in soft, dark, or pink sauerkraut. Without tasting it, discard the whole batch if it looks or smells as if it's gone bad.

Sauerkraut

Sauerkraut fermentation relies on salt to draw out the water in the cabbage; however, the salt isn't responsible for inhibiting the growth of undesirable bacteria, as some people might believe. Lactic acid bacteria are the force behind the fermentation.

2 pounds (900 g) cabbage, shredded or finely chopped
1 ounce (25 g) sea salt

Put the cabbage in a large bowl and sprinkle with the salt. Transfer to a fermenting crock (available from a fermentation supply company; see Sources, page 46) or a glass or food-grade plastic container. Press down the cabbage as you add it, forcing the juice out of the cabbage until the crock is full and the cabbage is covered by at least ½ inch of liquid. Put a food-grade weight (see Sources, page 46) or a sanitized stone on top of the cabbage to keep it submerged in the liquid.

Cover the container with a muslin cloth and let it sit in a cool place. If you're using a glass container, let the cabbage ferment in a dark area or cover the container with an opaque cloth. A brine will form in about 24 hours. Fermentation starts when bubbles of carbon dioxide begin to form and break through the surface of the brine.

Let the kraut ferment for at least 8 days, during which time the cabbage must remain submerged in the brine. A yeast bloom will develop on the surface of the liquid, creating a white layer. This is not harmful but should be removed every couple of days. Fermentation is complete when the bubbling ceases, depending on the ambient temperature. The best kraut is produced at 68 degrees F (20 degrees C).

Stored in a sealed container in the refrigerator, Sauerkraut will keep for 6 months.

Umeboshi

Umeboshi are small Japanese plums that are pickled in a 12 percent salt solution to which shiso leaves are added. The leaves add color, flavor, and, some people believe, medicinal benefits. The plums are pickled in the salt solution for six months. Traditionally produced umeboshi are high in sodium, although some producers are using less salt now that it's known that too much salt in the diet can lead to cardiovascular problems.

Beet Kvass (Sour Beet Juice)

Yield: 2 cups (500 ml)

This traditional beverage from eastern and some parts of central Europe is said to aid digestion. The kvass can be enjoyed as is or used as a base in borscht recipes. To get the full nutritional benefit of the kvass, serve it chilled or at room temperature to preserve the live microorganisms.

2 large or 4 medium beets, trimmed, scrubbed, and quartered
1 tablespoon (5 ml) sea salt

Put the beets in a sterilized 1-quart (1 L) glass jar, add the salt, and fill the jar with filtered water. Cover with a clean towel or cheesecloth and use a food-grade weight (available from a fermentation supply company; see Sources, page 46) or a sanitized stone to keep the beets submerged below the surface of the liquid during fermentation.

Let sit at room temperature (60 to 80 degrees F/16 to 27 degrees C) for 2 days or up to 2 weeks. Taste the liquid periodically. It should have a pleasant flavor and be slightly alcoholic. If the mixture smells bad, the beets have spoiled, and the mixture should be discarded.

When fermentation is complete, the kvass should have a salty sweet-and-sour taste and be slightly fizzy. Refrigerate when fermentation is complete. A gray yeast mold may form on top of the liquid. This is normal and will not affect the finished product. Simply skim it off before serving the kvass.

Rejuvelac

Yield: 8 cups (2 L)

This light fermented beverage can be enjoyed as is or used to make super-nutritious green smoothies or raw soups. This recipe is from *Sproutman's Kitchen Garden Cookbook* by Steve Meyerowitz.

½ cup (125 ml) soft wheat berries

Put the wheat berries in a small bowl. Cover with filtered water and let soak for 10 to 12 hours. Drain, rinse, and sprout for 3 days, rinsing and draining twice a day.

Put the sprouts in a blender with 3 cups of filtered water and process only until chopped; do not blend the sprouts. Pour into a sterilized 2-quart (2 L) glass jar, fill with filtered water, and cover the mouth of the jar with a muslin cloth. Let sit in a cool place (65 to 75 degrees F/18 to 24 degrees C) away from direct sunlight for 3 days. Stir the mixture twice a day, smelling it to make sure it seems fresh and hasn't developed an unpleasant aroma that would indicate spoilage.

After 3 days, taste some of the liquid; it should have a pleasant sour flavor similar to sauerkraut or sparkling lemon water. Stir and pour through a strainer to remove the sprouts. Reserve the sprouts to use for another batch.

Pour the remaining liquid into a jar, seal tightly, and refrigerate. Stored in the refrigerator, Rejuvelac will keep for 7 weeks. Remove the lid every 2 days to release the carbon dioxide buildup.

Acetic Acid Fermentation and Vinegar Production

The word vinegar is from the French term *vinaigre*, or sour wine. Its production is said to parallel that of winemaking, starting ten thousand years ago. Vinegar is made from fruit and vegetable juice, and the two-stage process

Cider Vinegar

Yield: 4 cups (1 L)

An essential ingredient for dressings and marinades, vinegar is a flavor powerhouse that offers the health benefits of a fermented food to boot.

Hard (alcoholic) apple cider
Unfiltered organic cider vinegar (or mother of vinegar)

Fill a sterilized 1-quart (1 L) widemouthed glass jar two-thirds with the hard apple cider. Pour in the cider vinegar until the jar is full (or add the mother of vinegar).

Cover the mouth of the jar with cheesecloth; vinegar fermentation is aerobic, so the substrate needs to be exposed to oxygen. Don't allow the cloth to touch the liquid.

Let the mixture sit in a dark place at room temperature (60 to 80 degrees F/16 to 27 degrees C) for 4 weeks. Do not disturb; if the mother of vinegar sinks to the bottom, the batch could be ruined. Taste occasionally to test if fermentation is complete; there should be no flavor of alcohol.

To store, pour the vinegar into bottles, being sure to fill the bottles all the way to the top. By leaving no air space, you create an anaerobic condition that will prevent spoilage.

involves yeasts and bacteria. Fermentation is initiated by yeasts, principally *Saccharomyces*, that break down the glucose in the juice to ethyl alcohol and carbon dioxide gas. Then *Acetobacter* bacteria break down the alcohol to acetic acid and water.

Vinegar can be made from a wide variety of raw materials, such as fruits, vegetables, and syrups, and these vary around the world, from the effervescent beverage kombucha to the palm wine vinegar found in Africa and east Asia. In vinegar production, these raw materials must first undergo alcoholic fermentation, similar to wine production. Vinegar can also be made directly from wine; in fact, the best raw materials for vinegar are hard apple cider and wine. When finished, high-quality vinegar should have an acidic acid strength of around 6 percent.

The microorganisms involved in making vinegar grow at the top of the liquid, forming a jelly-like mass known as the "mother of vinegar." The mother is composed of both yeasts and bacteria that work together to convert the substrate into vinegar. The important yeasts in this process are *Saccharomyces cerevisiae* and *S. ellipsoideus.* The important bacteria are *Acetobacter aceti, A. ascendens, and A. xylinum*. Strong vinegar is often added to the liquid substrate at the beginning of the fermentation process to encourage the growth of *Acetobacter* bacteria and discourage the establishment of undesirable microorganisms.

Foods and Beverages Produced by Bacteria, Yeast, and Mold Combinations

Like bacteria, yeasts and molds are found throughout nature, in the air, the soil, and the intestinal tracts of animals and humans. These microorganisms are instrumental in the making of basic foods, such as breads and alcoholic beverages.

Foods

Certain foods rely on more than one type of microorganism for fermentation. These include leavened breads (including sourdough bread) and tempeh, a plant-based form of protein.

Leavened and Sourdough Bread

Fermentation is caused by the action of a symbiotic colony of bacteria and yeasts (often referred to by the acronym SCOBY) that works interdependently to process different nutrients in the substrate. In the making of sourdough bread, for example, a combination of lactobacilli and a starter culture of indigenous wild yeast is used. Common wild yeasts used are *Kazachstania exigua* and *Saccharomyces cerevisiae.*

In general, in the making of leavened breads, wheat or rye flour, water, and yeast are mixed and kneaded to form bread dough. The yeast produces carbon dioxide that gets trapped in the sticky dough and causes it to rise. The dough is allowed to rise for a time and then baked. The semihard crust formed during baking is a deterrent to spoilage bacteria. Leavened breads are popular in Europe, the Middle East, and North America.

Injera

Injera is a spongy Ethiopian flatbread made from teff flour that's sometimes mixed with wheat flour. The flour is mixed with water and allowed to ferment naturally with wild yeast for one to three days. If the mixture doesn't ferment, some baker's yeast may be added. When it's ready, the batter is cooked in a hot, oiled skillet, just as pancakes are cooked.

Tempeh

Tempeh is a soybean cake and an important food product that has been used for centuries in Indonesia and Malaysia. It's a nutritious, high-protein food and can be used as a meat substitute in stir-fries and other dishes. The mold used for fermentation is *Rhizopus oligosporus* or a related *Rhizopus* species that occurs naturally in the region of production. The substrate is partially cooked soybeans that have been soaked, dehulled, and split.

During soaking, lactic acid fermentation occurs as a result of the naturally present *Lactobacillus* bacteria, decreasing the pH to 5 or below and inhibiting the growth of spoilage organisms. The *Rhizopus* molds aren't affected by the acid environment, so they proliferate.

During fermentation, the *Rhizopus* culture knits the split soybeans into a compact cake, and a fine white plume of mold covers its surface. When fermentation is complete, the soybean cakes are removed from the liquid, spread out in thin sheets, and surface-dried. Drying further inhibits the growth of spoilage bacteria. The raw tempeh is then ready for use and must be cooked for fifteen minutes before eating.

In the United States and other temperate regions, soaking does not produce the natural lactic acid fermentation and lower pH that inhibits the growth of unwanted bacteria. In this situation, *Lactobacillus plantarum* bacteria or vinegar is added to the soaking water to create the necessary acid environment.

Beverages

Since ancient times, yeast fermentation has been used to make alcoholic beverages. Any fruit or sweet plant sap can be fermented to produce an alcoholic beverage. For example, grape wine is important in Algeria, Argentina, Chile, France, Georgia, Morocco, South Africa, and the United States. In Africa, banana beer is a popular alcoholic fruit drink. Other fruits used to make alcoholic drinks include dates in North Africa, pineapples in Latin America, and jackfruit in Asia.

Beer and Wine

Beer is made from a mixture of mashed grains (barley, wheat, and rye), hops, and yeast. In addition, a variety of flavors are often added. When wine is made, grapes are crushed and combined with cultured yeast or wild yeast that occurs naturally on the grapes. The mixture is allowed to ferment, then is aged in wooden barrels. The whole process is called vinification and produces wine with an alcoholic content of 10 to 14 percent. In both beer and wine production, the species of yeast used is *Saccharomyces cerevisiae.*

Hard Cider

Fresh apple cider without any preservatives provides the best foundation for hard cider. Often a starter culture is used to ensure that fermentation will begin. The common yeast for fermentation is *Saccharomyces uvarum*. The cider and yeast mixture ferments at 60 to 70 degrees F (16 to 21 degrees C) for about two weeks. Once the bubbling stops, primary fermentation is complete, and the cider must sit for another week to allow the yeast to settle out. After that the yeast sediment is carefully removed, and the cider is bottled and allowed to sit for another two weeks before it's ready to drink.

Kombucha

Hailed as "the tea of immortality," kombucha has ancient origins; in fact, its use was first recorded in East Asia in 221 BC. Also known as Manchurian mushroom tea, the fermented drink is not made from a mushroom but rather relies on a symbiotic colony of bacteria and yeasts (SCOBY) for fermentation. The main components that produce the SCOBY are *Acetobacter xylinum* bacteria and *Saccharomyces cerevisiae* and *Schizosaccharomyces pombe* yeasts. Their interaction produces a spongy, somewhat slimy, brown, solid, rubbery disk (to some, perhaps, resembling a large, flat mushroom) called "the mother." In addition, the making of kombucha is dependent on oxygen.

The bacteria in the mother produces acetic acid and glucuronic acid; the yeast produces alcohol and carbonation. Depending on how long the fermentation is allowed to continue, some batches of kombucha can contain an alcohol content of 1 to 3 percent.

Kombucha tea has a sweet-sour taste, similar to apple cider, and is slightly carbonated. Said to have many health benefits, it's considered a biological food with antiviral and antibiotic properties and no negative side effects. Commercial kombucha is pasteurized, so it doesn't contain healthful, live microorganisms like the home-brewed version.

Kombucha

Yield: 8 cups (2 L)

Making kombucha is a simple process and can be easily done in your kitchen once you have a SCOBY to start it with. This recipe is adapted from *Kombucha Rediscovered* by Klaus Kaufmann.

8 cups (2 L) filtered water
1 cup (250 ml) sugar
4 bags black tea, or 3½ tablespoons (52 ml) loose black tea
3 tablespoons (45 ml) kombucha tea from a previous batch or the liquid the SCOBY came in
Kombucha SCOBY

Bring the water to a boil in a stainless steel pot. Remove from the heat, add the sugar, and stir to completely dissolve. Add the tea bags or loose tea and let steep for 10 to 15 minutes. Remove the tea bags or strain out the tea leaves. Let the tea cool to lukewarm.

Add the kombucha tea or SCOBY liquid and transfer to a large glass bowl, ideally one that has a lid. Don't use a metal pot. Gently transfer the SCOBY to the liquid in the bowl, making sure the lighter, smoother side is facing up. The SCOBY will float on top of the liquid.

Cover the bowl with the lid or a white cotton cloth. Don't let the cloth touch the liquid or SCOBY. Put the bowl in a well-ventilated location where it won't be disturbed. It should be kept away from direct sunlight and at room temperature (60 to 80 degrees F/16 to 27 degrees C); it also should be kept away from potted plants and any area that could contain mold. Let the tea ferment for 7 to 14 days. The shorter time produces a sweeter tea; the longer time produces a more sour tea.

A new kombucha SCOBY may have formed by the time fermentation is complete. When the kombucha has fermented to your taste, transfer the SCOBY or SCOBYs from the bowl to another clean glass bowl. Pour the kombucha into glass bottles and top with corks or loose-fitting lids. Be sure to save 1 cup of tea for your next batch.

Store the kombucha in the refrigerator for up to 2 weeks. Even though fermentation is slowed down appreciably by refrigeration, the drink will continue to ferment. So use caution when opening kombucha; a bottle might forcefully pop its cork.

Koji

Cultivated since ancient times in the Far East, Koji is a fermented product made from a combination of bacteria and fungi in rice, barley, or soybeans. It is the basis for such drinks and condiments as miso, rice vinegar, sake, shochu (spirits), and shoyu.

In the koji culture, the predominant types of bacteria are *Staphylococcus* and *Weissella*, and the predominant fungi are *Aspergillus* and *Candida*. The word "koji" can refer to either the fungus (*Aspergillus oryzae)* or the final fermented product. In 2006, koji was designated a "national fungus" by the Brewing Society of Japan because of its importance in fermented food production.

While Japanese cuisine relies heavily on koji-based condiments, such as miso and shoyu, many other Asian nations depend on their own versions of salty and savory sauces and pastes—soy sauce in China and kecap in Malaysia.

Probiotics

Experts from the Food and Agricultural Organization of the United Nations and the World Health Organization define probiotics as "live microorganisms which, when administered in adequate amounts, confer a health benefit on the host." Two of the most widely studied types of probiotics are *Bifidobacterium* and *Lactobacillus*.

Probiotics can be acquired by eating fermented food products like those described in this book or by taking a probiotic supplement. Not to be confused with probiotics, *prebiotics* are nondigestible, fermentable food products that stimulate the growth and activity of beneficial bacteria. They are, in essence, food for the microbiota. The sugar in these foods cannot be broken down by gastric juices, so it makes its way through the stomach and into the intestines, where the microbiota feeds on it. Some whole foods, such as artichokes, asparagus, bananas, chicory, garlic, Jerusalem artichokes, leeks, legumes (beans, peas, and lentils), onions, and sweet potatoes, naturally contain prebiotics. In addition, prebiotics are sold in supplement form.

Like prebiotics, probiotics are sold as dietary supplements. Proponents of probiotic supplements claim they're effective for the treatment of a whole host of ailments and health conditions (see box, page 39). However, at present, there's no scientific evidence to support these claims. The Federal Drug Administration and the European Food Safety Authority haven't as yet approved any health claims for probiotic supplements. Despite this fact, millions of people use them every day. Probiotic supplements are a big business, and yearly sales may surpass one billion dollars in the near future. This may happen sooner rather than later depending on what the research tells us: many studies involving probiotics have been funded by manufacturers in the last ten years in an effort to lend scientific credibility to their health claims.

For now we must rely on preliminary studies done mostly on animals and some on humans, along with anecdotal reports that strongly indicate that the oral ingestion of probiotic supplements is helpful for a wide range of disorders both inside and outside the gastrointestinal tract. A study published in the *Journal of Applied Microbiotics* stated the following: "The way probiotics bring about their beneficial effects is largely unknown but is thought to be caused by a number of factors: modifying gut pH, suppressing pathogens by the production of antimicrobial compounds, competing with pathogens for living space and available nutrients and growth factors, and by stimulating the immune system."

Health Benefits of Probiotics

Probiotics have been shown to be helpful for people with the following conditions:

- bacterial vaginosis
- cancer
- childhood allergies and intestinal inflammation disorders
- diarrhea associated with antibiotic treatment
- *Helicobacter pylori* infections (this bacteria causes stomach ulcers)
- high cholesterol
- hypertension or high blood pressure
- inflammatory bowel disease, irritable bowel syndrome, and ulcerative colitis
- lactose intolerance
- recurrent thrush
- rheumatoid arthritis
- urinary tract infections

Probiotics are also believed to do the following:

- benefit radiation treatment patients
- defend the host from pathogens
- improve dental health
- improve intestinal health
- provide a limited protection against heart disease
- protect foreign travelers against food poisoning and diarrhea
- rebuild and maintain the composition and diversity of gut microbiota
- stimulate immune system activity
- synthesize and enhance the bioavailability of nutrients
- synthesize certain vitamins

Microorganism Strains in Probiotics

The human gastrointestinal tract contains as many as five hundred different microbial species. The two most common are *Lactobacillus acidophilus* and *Bifidobacterium bifidum*, which are also the main bacteria found in probiotic supplements. *Enterococcus, Lactococcus, and Streptococcus* species are also included in some formulas. Each probiotic bacteria can produce specific health effects (see "Advantages of Specific Microorganism Strains," below). Probiotic supplement labels usually list the genus, species, and strain they contain. A little online research will tell you which strains produce the health effects you're interested in. Overall, it's recommended that you choose a product that contains multiple species rather than just one.

In the United States there is no national standard for the number or species of microorganisms that must be in a probiotic formula. Manufacturers aren't required to list this information, but there are some who do. Generally, the dose for children should be 5 to 10 billion colony-forming units (CFU) per day, and the dose for adults should be 10 to 20 billion CFU per day per day.

Most probiotic supplements can be found in the refrigerated section of the vitamin and supplement department of most health food stores, although some formulations don't require refrigeration. Preparations come in the form of capsules, pastes, powders, sprays, or tablets, and certain forms are preferred depending on the condition being treated. Probiotic supplements do have expiration dates, after which time they're no longer guaranteed to be active.

Advantages of Specific Microorganism Strains

Research has shown that certain health conditions respond to specific strains of microorganisms. As a result, probiotic supplement manufacturers have developed formulations to target specific health conditions.

Bifidobacterium. This bacteria reduces the incidence of neonatal necrotizing enterocolitis, a bacterial infection in newborns that causes part of the intestines to die.

Enterococcus faecium. This bacteria decreases the duration of acute diarrhea caused by gastroenteritis, the inflammation of the stomach and intestines.

Lactobacillus acidophilus. This bacteria offers multiple benefits. It improves the digestion of lactose, which decreases the incidence of diarrhea and the other symptoms of lactose intolerance. It also ameliorates diarrhea in children and individuals with short-bowel syndrome. In addition, it reduces inflammation of the ileal pouch, an artificial rectum surgically created out of ileal gut tissue in patients who have undergone a colectomy. *Lactobacillus acidophilus* also is used in microbial interference therapy, which is the use of nonpathogenic bacteria to eliminate pathogens and as an adjunct to antibiotics. And finally, this bacteria improves mucosal immune function and mucin secretion, which aid in the prevention of disease.

Lactobacillus plantarum. This bacteria has been shown to reduce the incidence of diarrhea in children enrolled in day-care centers. It's also especially effective in reducing inflammation and pain in people with inflammatory bowel syndrome, small bowel bacterial overgrowth in children, bloating, and flatulence. In addition, this bacteria has shown a positive effect on immunity in children with HIV.

Lactobacillus reuteri. This bacteria shortens the duration of acute gastroenteritis, or infectious diarrhea.

Lactobacillus rhamnosus. In a controlled trial, this bacteria enhanced cellular immunity in healthy adults.

Lactobacillus salivarius. As a result of the lactic acid they secrete, this bacteria suppressed and eradicated *Helicobacter pylori*, the bacteria that causes stomach ulcers, in tissue cultures and animal models.

Bacteroides. This bacteria has positive effects on arthritis, chronic colitis, and gastritis. In studies, it was shown to increase bacterial urease activity in chronic juvenile arthritis.

Saccharomyces boulardii. This yeast reduces the recurrence of diarrhea caused by *Clostridium difficile*. In studies involving the bacteria *C. difficile* and *Klebsiella oxytoca*, this yeast decreased the risk and shortened the duration of antibiotic-associated diarrhea, shortened the duration of acute gastroenteritis, and decreased functional diarrhea but not any other symptoms of irritable bowel syndrome.

Possible Probiotic Side Effects

There have been no reports of infections caused by probiotics, but infection is a possibility for people taking certain strains. People who are critically ill or those with a weakened immune system, such as cancer patients receiving chemotherapy, should avoid probiotics. People who are hospitalized or need heart valve surgery should avoid probiotics because of the risk of infection. Probiotic use may make children more likely to experience allergies.

Research

Through microscopic analysis, we know that the microbial cells living in association with humans number in the billions and, until recently, this vast and diverse community of microorganisms has remained largely unstudied. Not much is known about its influence on human development, physiology, immunity, and nutrition.

That's beginning to change with the formation of the National Institutes of Health (NIH) Human Microbiome Project (HMP). According to the organization, HMP "was established with the mission of generating research resources enabling comprehensive characterization of the human microbiota and analysis of its role in human health and disease."

Because of the recent developments in the field of biology, researchers can now look at the metabolic capabilities encoded in the genes of microbial communities and begin to understand the influence they have on human physiology and disease. These advancements include genomics, which involves applying the techniques of genetics and molecular biology to genetic mapping and DNA sequencing; transcriptomics, the use of biomarkers to test drug safety; and the study of proteins, metabolites, and the interactions of molecules in cells.

As part of this effort, the HMP has created the first genome sequencing reference database and has identified between 81 and 99 percent of all types of microorganisms living on and in healthy adults. HMP researchers estimate that more than ten thousand microbial species live within the human ecosystem and that they contribute some eight million genes to our 22,000 genes.

"We now have a very good idea of what is normal for a healthy Western population and are beginning to learn how changes in the microbiome correlate with physiology and disease," said James M. Anderson, MD, one of the directors of HMP.

NIH has funded medical studies using this data and acknowledged in a 2012 press release the role the microbiota plays in multiple health conditions. These include Crohn's disease, ulcerative colitis, and esophageal cancer; skin microbiome in psoriasis and immunodeficiency; urogenital microbiome in reproductive and sexual history and circumcision; and a number of childhood disorders, including pediatric abdominal pain, intestinal inflammation, and enterocolitis, a severe condition in premature infants in which a part of the intestines actually dies.

There have been some interesting and unexpected findings from the research. For example, scientists have discovered that almost everyone carries microbes in their gut that cause illnesses. In healthy people, these microbes cause no disease; they live in peaceful coexistence with their host and other members of the gut microbiome. What researchers want to know is why and under what conditions these pathogens sometimes turn deadly. This knowledge could revise the thinking about how microorganisms cause disease.

Another unexpected finding is that in the human gut there are certain bacteria that assist the digestion of carbohydrates, fats, and proteins. It turns out that the same specific species of bacteria may not always be metabolizing these compounds. Rather, it appears that bacteria species can actually swap metabolic function.

Researchers also found that the composition of the human microbiome changes over time. For instance, during illness or antibiotic treatment, the microbes in a person's gut may change substantially according to how the microbes are affected. The gut microbiome eventually returns to a state of equilibrium when the stress is abated, but not necessarily with the same species composition.

The data collected in this NIH effort has been made available to researchers around the world and will stimulate advances in infectious disease research that would have been impossible without it.

Conclusion

As we have learned, microbes are present literally everywhere in our environment: the air, soil, rocks, sea, and so on. And there is constant competition between them, and between them and us, for available food. Microbes left alone mostly spoil food, making it unfit to eat. In a typical home kitchen, many pounds of rotten fruit and vegetables are discarded throughout the year.

However, a number of microbes are beneficial to food production and under controlled conditions produce desirable fermented food products. These items offer appealing flavors, aromas, and textures; increased nutritional value; and significant health benefits. The craft of making fermented food is all about how to make these microbes work to our advantage. The fermentation process is, in effect, controlled spoilage.

Fermentation, as we now know, is a process in which enzymes produced by microorganisms break down carbohydrates, fats, and proteins into simpler compounds. This makes fermented food easier to digest, increases its nutritional value, and eliminates toxins.

Under the right conditions, fruits and some vegetables naturally ferment by the action of wild microbes that are living on their skins. Fruit juice can ferment to wine, and wine can turn to vinegar. Cabbage, with a little added salt, can ferment to sauerkraut by the actions of the wild microbes living on its leaves. Raw milk ferments from naturally occurring microbes and can be used in baking to improve the flavor and texture of bread. If the whey is allowed to evaporate, a simple cheese is the result.

There is solid scientific evidence that humans have been intentionally producing fermented beverages since Neolithic times, the period during which cereal cultivation and animal domestication were introduced. Since then, mostly by trial and error, we have discovered how to produce a wide array of fermented foods and beverages.

Even though fermented foods had been consumed for centuries the world over, it was not until the 1800s, through the work of Louis Pasteur and others, that we began to understand the underlying process at work. During this period, scientists discovered that fermentation was caused by the actions of enzymes produced by microorganisms.

Humans couldn't exist without the symbiotic relationship we have with the tens of millions of friendly microorganisms that inhabit each of our bodies. They're involved in many metabolic functions and help to keep us healthy. The ones that live in the gut are involved in digestion, protect us from pathogens, boost our immune function, and do much, much more. At the same time, there are pathogenic microorganisms that live within us, and given the right conditions, they can quickly multiply and make us sick. So it's important to keep a healthy balance of microbes in our systems. Consuming fermented foods helps maintain this microbial balance.

Long used in other parts of the world, fermented foods have become popular in the West as more people experience both their culinary rewards and the many health benefits they offer. An increasing number of people have experienced the joy and satisfaction of producing these foods at home in their own kitchens. It's not hard to do. Many fermented foods can be produced with basic equipment. So go ahead and include fermented foods in your diet, and eat a serving each day. You might just enjoy a long and healthy life as a result of doing so.

Sources

Fermentation Supplies and Crocks

Cultures for Health

culturesforhealth.com

Harvest Essentials

harvestessentials.com

Fermentation Groups

Many online groups exist; the following two offer a lot of good information.

Fermenters Club

fermentersclub.com

This community of food enthusiasts shares a love for traditionally preserved, natural probiotic foods.

Google+ Group

Cultured/Fermented Foods

This community is all about cultured and fermented foods and beverages.

Medical Information

American Society for Microbiology

asm.org

The Human Microbiome Project

nih.gov

uBiome

ubiome.com

This company provides test kits and results that allow you to learn more about your microbiome with DNA sequencing.

References

Bates, Dorothy. 1989. *The Tempeh Cookbook*. Summertown, TN: Book Publishing Company.

Battcock, Mike, and Sue Azam-Ali. 1998. *Fermented Fruits and Vegetables: A Global Perspective*. Food and Agriculture Organization of the United Nations, Rome. fao.org/docrep/x0560e/x0560e00.htm.

Davis, Brenda, and Vesanto Melina. 2013. *Becoming Vegan: Express Edition*. Summertown, TN: Book Publishing Company.

Funkhouser, L. J., and S. R. Bordenstein. 2013. "Mom Knows Best: The Universality of Maternal Microbial Transmission." *PLOS Biol* 11(8): e1001631. Doi: 10.1371/journal.pbio.1001631.

Holzapfel, Cynthia. 2002. *Apple Cider Vinegar for Weight Loss and Good Health*. Summertown, TN: Healthy Living Publications.

Islami, F., J. Ren, and F. Kamangar. 2009. "Pickled Vegetables and the Risk of Esophageal Cancer: A Meta-analysis. *British Journal of Cancer*. 101: 1641–1647. Doi: 10.1038/sj.bjc.6605372.

Kaufman, Klaus. 2013. *Kombucha Rediscovered*. Summertown, TN: Books Alive.

Kaufman, Klaus. 2008. *Making Sauerkraut and Pickled Vegetables at Home*. Summertown, TN: Books Alive.

McDougall, John. 2006. *Dr. McDougall's Digestive Tune-Up*. Summertown, TN: Healthy Living Publications.

Meyerowitz, Steve. 1999. *Sproutman's Kitchen Garden Cookbook*. Barrington, MA: Sproutman Publications.

National Institutes of Health. Human Microbiome Project. http://commonfund.nih.gov/hmp/index.

Parvez, S., et al. 2006. "Probiotics and Their Fermented Food Products Are Beneficial for Health." *Journal of Applied Microbiology*. 100(6): 1171–1185.

Selhub, Eva, Alan Logan, and Alison Bested. 2014. "Fermented Food, Microbiota, and Mental Health: Ancient Practice Meets Nutritional Psychiatry." *Journal of Physiological Anthropology*. Jan. 15 (33): 2.

Shurtleff, William, and Akido Aoyagi. 2007. *History of Soybeans and Soyfoods: 1100 BC to the 1980s*. Lafayette, CA: Soyinfo Center. Unpublished.

Steinkraus, K. H. 2002. "Fermentations in World Food Processing." *Comprehensive Reviews in Food Science and Food Safety*. 1(1): 23–32.

Todar, Kenneth. *Todar's Online Textbook of Bacteriology*. textbookofbacteriology.net.